Candida:

10 Lessons That Will Teach You How To Minimize Discomfort And Cure Yeast Infections Quickly

Table of content

Candida: 1

    10 Lessons That Will Teach You How To Minimize Discomfort And Cure Yeast Infections
    Quickly..1

Introduction 3

Chapter 1 – Candida: An Overview 5

Chapter 2 – Causes and Diagnoses of Candida 9

Chapter 3 – The Ten Easiest Ways To Treat Candida Naturally 14

Chapter 4 – Candida Diet: Keeping It Real 20

Chapter 5 – The Healthy Life: Candida Where it Should Be 25

Conclusion 28

Introduction

Bacteria.

It's all around us.

We see soaps that are anti-bacterial. We see commercials that tell us there's bacteria all around us, in the air we breathe, the doors, carts, or other items we touch, and even in the food we eat. If we have a diagnoses from the doctor, it will usually specify whether it is bacterial or not.

You see charts about the little guys, you see billboards about them, and you even see them appear in different tv shows for a variety of reason, but the information about them is vastly different for something that looks just like all the others.

You are told that you want good bacteria in your stomach, then you are told to avoid a certain kind of bacteria or you will get sick. You are told that there are bacteria all around you, then you are told that you want to avoid the stuff for health and sanitation purposes.

You want it, you don't.

So what do you do?

The answer is to get smart. If you experience bad breath, a white tongue, yeast infections anywhere on your body, headaches, or countless other symptoms, the actual culprit may surprise you, as so many people blame this on bacteria, when it is actually a form of fungus known as candida.

Don't be alarmed, though the word *fungus* can be scary, this can be completely managed, taken care of, or prevented all by a few simple things you can do without ever setting foot inside a doctor's office? That's right, you can treat and cure a number of issues in a variety of ways that I am going to show you, and you can prevent it from coming back with a diet that is so easy to follow, anyone can do it.

So are you ready to get rid of those symptoms and embrace a healthy life? Are you ready say goodbye to those things every coming back and bothering you again?

If you are, read on, because this book is going to change everything for you in ways that are so easy, you will wonder why you never did it before.

What are you waiting for?

Chapter 1 – Candida: An Overview

Odds are, if you are reading this book, you are experiencing candida in some way. You may feel embarrassed about it, you may feel some discomfort, or you may just want to get it under control.

Right now, you may be feeling stressed, just wanting to get this taken care of quickly, without having to worry about it coming back. I know how you feel, and I am going to help you get there, but first, I want you to understand what candida is, and the symptoms it can bring about.

The first step to fixing anything is understanding it, and that includes things that involve your health. If you want to get rid of this for good, you need to understand what it is first of all, then we will focus on how to get rid of it, then how to keep it from coming back again.

Candida is a fungus

The reason the main symptom of candida is because candida itself is a fungus... or, more specifically, a yeast. That knowledge in itself can add some comfort to a lot of people, knowing that it is only a variety of yeast that can easily be controlled.

Where does it comes from, and how did I get this in me?

Candida is not contagious, you didn't catch it from someone, and you didn't get it from using something that was contaminated. Everyone on the planet has candida in several places internally. When you experience these symptoms, you are experiencing an overgrowth of this fungus in your body.

You can think of it as any other bodily ailment that comes from within, whether it be indigestion, heartburn, or acid reflux. Our naturally produce all kinds of things, but when they get out of hand, we start to experience symptoms.

If candida is inside of everyone, then why do we have it?

When it is working normally, the main job of candida is to help in the absorption of food in the body. This is actually a really good thing, as it's what keeps us functioning at our best.

That's when things get tricky. You want to have enough of this fungus in your body, but when you get too much of it, you are going to experience the symptoms that you don't want to have. These symptoms have such a wide range, it can be hard to pinpoint candida as the issue right at first.

Thankfully, there are several solutions to too much candida, and you can easily manage your levels through natural lifestyle changes, no doctors or prescriptions involved.

What kind of symptoms can candida cause in the body?

If you have a candida overgrowth, you may experience a variety of symptoms. These may be as simple as one or two, or you may have quite of few on the list. Check these out and see if you are experiencing any of them.

- Fungal problems on the skin or nails, which can include athlete's foot

- Always feeling tired or worn out, even when you haven't been busy or active

- Problems with digestion including diarrhea, bloating, or stomach cramps

- Poor memory or having a tough time concentrating on what you are doing… this can be in varying degrees, so keep an eye out

- Skin issues

- Mood issues, whether those be mood swings, irritability, anxiety, or even depression in some cases

- Vaginal or urinary tract problems, including rashes, yeast infections, or rectal itching

- Cravings for junk foods containing refined carbs or a lot of sugars

- Allergies, especially of the skin and itchy ears

- Mouth issues, such as bad breath or coated tongue

- Oral thrush

Of course, this isn't a complete list of the signs and symptoms, but you can see here that there are many different ways this can manifest itself in your body. If you are experiencing one or more of the symptoms on the list, don't worry that there is something horribly wrong, because it's more than likely you are dealing with a candida overgrowth.

This can happen to anyone, and in reality, it is rather common. The good news is that it's easy to diagnose, cure, and prevent.

Chapter 2 – Causes and Diagnoses of Candida

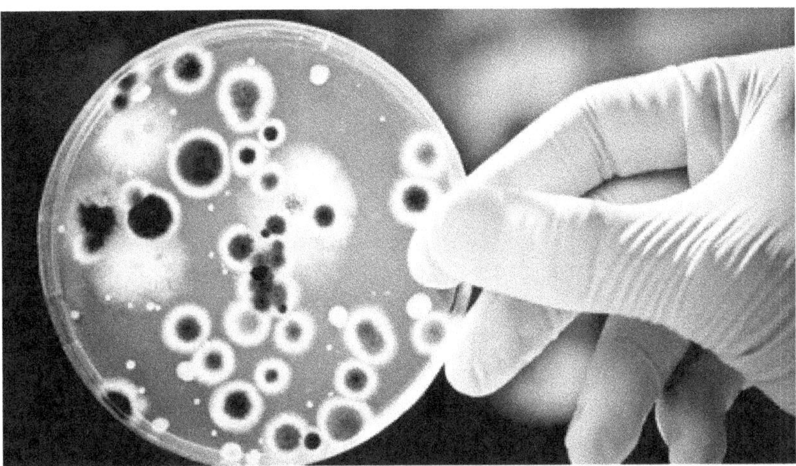

As I said in the last chapter, everyone has some candida in them at all times, this is because it is something that we need to function properly, and digest our food. When you get an overgrowth, you are going to experience the symptoms listed in the previous chapter, which means this is relatively easy to diagnose.

With that in mind, I'm sure you are wondering what causes this, and how to know for sure if you do, in fact, have it.

What causes Candida overgrowth?

Ironically enough, candida overgrowth is largely caused by what you eat. This makes sense since you know that its natural function in your body is to aid in digestion. If you take a moment to examine your diet, you are going to likely find that you are guilty of one or more of these, which are certain to be the culprits in the overgrowth.

On the plus side, diet is one of the easiest things you can change about yourself, and after we determine what the problem is, we are going to be able to easily determine how you can fix it.

- Alcohol consumption – unfortunately, this is one of the biggest culprits in this problem. It doesn't actually matter how much you drink, if you do drink, you are at risk for developing this overgrowth

- Eating a lot of foods with refined carbs and that are high in sugar – this is by far the biggest issue many people face in their overgrowth. The standard diets these days hold many foods that are both full of refined carbs and high in sugars.

  In the chapters to come, I am going to show you which foods these are help you learn how to avoid them

- Eating a diet that is high in the beneficial foods – I know it sounds confusing at first, but even foods such as sauerkraut and kombucha can be culprits when it comes to candida overgrowth, which I will also explain better later on

- Oral contraceptives – this is one thing a lot of women don't want to give up, but don't worry, you aren't going to have to and you can still control this problem, I just want you to be aware of all the possible causes

- Killing too many of your good bacteria can also cause this problem – our body is like a machine full of other organisms working together to make things happen, but if your system gets out of balance, even with itself, you may experience this kind of overgrowth.

This can be done quite easily, if you are on antibiotics for one reason or another, you could see this happen quickly. Again, the benefit of the diet I am going to outline for you is going to get rid of this problem and return your body to the balance you want.

As you can see by this list, it is incredibly easy to get an overgrowth in your system. You can even live a healthy life and see this happen, so don't worry that you caused it by doing something you shouldn't be.

The problem with candida is that it takes advantage of the foods you put into your body, so if you are eating or drinking too much of one thing, and there isn't enough good bacteria to keep it in check, you are going to get the overgrowth, which is going to lead to those symptoms I listed before.

I am sure by looking at the list of symptoms and the list of causes, you are able to pretty accurately diagnose this in yourself or a loved one,

but if you did want to go to the doctor to check for sure, here is what you can expect:

Some people are comfortable with their own diagnoses and treatments, and the good news is, you can accurately and effectively take care of this without ever setting foot inside a doctor's office.

On the other hand, there are people who really like to have the peace of mind of going into the doctor's office, and getting an official diagnoses from there. If you are going to do this, here is what you can expect to happen.

- **Testing** – of course the only way to see if you have an overgrowth through a doctor's office is through testing of some kind, and you are going to get the option to do one or more of several kinds.

  There are blood tests in which they take a small sample, or there are times when you may take a stool sample. There are even urine samples and testing they can do, so you have plenty of options.

- **Your doctor will run the tests and get back to you** – depending on the office you are in, this can be within minutes or it could take a couple of days. Either way, once you have your diagnoses, you are going to be given a list of treatment options that are much the same as what I am going to outline for you in the next couple chapters.

Is there a medication I can take for this?

As with most things these days, there is a medication you can take, but this is only going to jump start your treatment, as your doctor is going to recommend you change your diet and focus on the ways you can prevent this naturally.

As I have said before, you can go to the doctor if you want the official report, but I have found that this is much easier (and less expensive) to handle on your own, and you can be certain that you are getting the same results you would be if you want in to have it taken care of.

So let's turn our attention now from the causes and effect of this to the treatment and prevention, which, of course, is the main reason we are here anyway.

Chapter 3 – The Ten Easiest Ways To Treat Candida Naturally

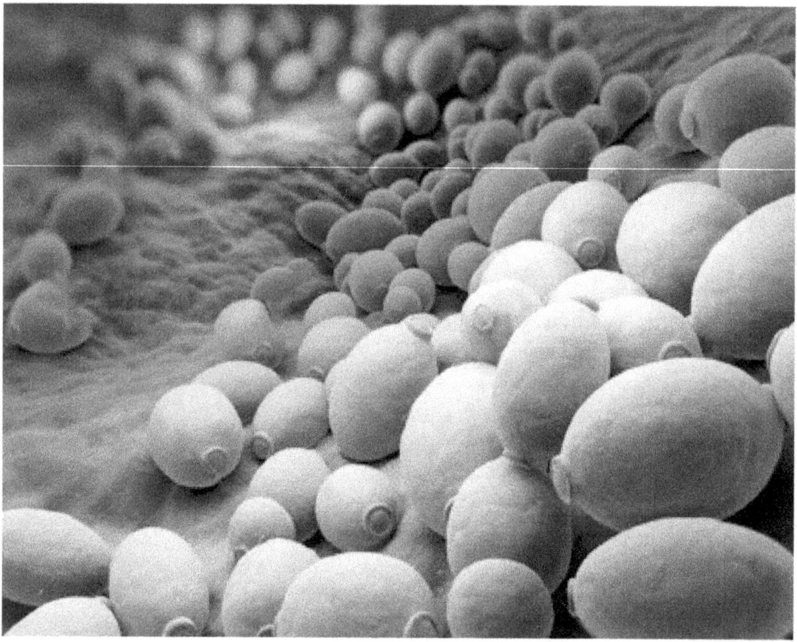

Truly, there's no doctor visits or medications required when you follow these simple and easy cures, and you are going to find that they are painless, not at all embarrassing, and inexpensive, the best way to treat anything, after all.

1. **Stop feeding the problem** – yeast loves sugar, and if you are putting things into your body that is going to feed this, you are only feeding the problem.

Remember that diets high in sugary foods are only making this worse, and if you drink alcohol, remember that alcohol is changed into sugar in your body... which is only feeding the candida. Stop the feeding, starve the problem.

2. **Cut out the refined carbs as much as you can** – again, feeding the problem is only going to work against you in the long run, and if you are eating things with a lot of refined carbs, you are only putting more and more food into your body for the yeast to feed on, which is going to make it a lot harder to get rid of.

3. **Make war on the problem** – I am sure by now you have realized that this stuff is alive, after all, if you are feeding it and it is growing, it is clearly something that is alive and functioning, making it something you can actively fight.

Candida can be fought in a variety of ways, but I find such things as grapeseed oil to be highly effective. Simply add a few drops to your tea a few times a month, and watch the victory be yours.

4. **Balance out the numbers** – your body is an entire system of live beings all working together to function properly. If you want to make sure your candida population stays where it should be, you need to make sure your numbers stay the same all over your body.

To do this, keep your populations of the other bacteria at the right amount, and your body is going to regulate everything as it should. Remember that there are certain things such as antibiotics that will kill off the good bacteria, and there are foods that will replace these as well (think yogurt and other fermented foods like that)

5. **Remember though, balance in everything is the key to success –** what you are experiencing is a candida overgrowth, another way to say this is that your body has gotten out of whack with itself, and as such it is growing too much of one thing and not enough of the other.

When you are restoring your body to natural balance, you want it to be in natural balance, which means you don't want to overdo the battle on candida. It is helpful in its own right, so don't put in too much oil or yogurt to get rid of it, stay with normal servings daily and you will be fine.

6. **Keep your stress levels at bay –** again with the balance system. One of the causes of candida that I didn't list up above is stress. Stress can be behind so many issues it can be hard to pinpoint as being responsible for other things such as this, but trust me, if you are stressing about getting this under control, you are, in fact, making it harder to get under control.

Ease up on your stress and do things that release it, such as yoga, taking walks, or meditation. You are going to benefit from it in more ways than one if you engage in any of these activities, and your candida is going to get back to where it should be, too.

7. **Detox your body regularly, keeping everything where it should be** – too many people get lazy when it comes to their health, until they start to see things in their body go wrong. You don't want this to be normal for you, so work on keeping it at bay.

   Regularly detox your body through any method you like, whether you do juice detoxes, water cleanses, or veggie cleanses. Make sure you are going with the natural foods and that you focus on real, healthy foods. Again, you could potentially do more harm than good if you go back to eating out of balance with yourself.

8. **Water is your best friend, and so is great hygiene-** I don't want you to misunderstand with this, you don't get a candida overgrowth through poor hygiene, but I can assure you that you will see it reduce itself dramatically if you are careful to instill good hygiene routines into your day.

   Drink lots of water all throughout your day, keeping your body well hydrated and flushes of toxins, and in addition, make sure you are doing things such as brushing your tongue with your scrub brush, washing your hands and feet and drying them thoroughly, making sure your creases and folds are clean and dry, free of anything that will promote yeast growth.

   These are things that take some getting used to, especially if you are already a clean person, and it doesn't feel like you need to take steps to be cleaner, but let me assure you, the less friendly your body is to the growth of this candida, the less likely it is will be to overgrow.

9. **Maintain a well-balanced life on the inside and out** – think of this as a combination of the last two steps. You don't want to let stress take over your life, but you also want to make sure that you regularly engage in things that make you happy.

You would be surprised to know how many things in life come not from too much of something, but from a lack of something else. In other words, you may do your best to de-stress through your day, but unless you are replacing this stress with something positive, you are going to deal with this all over again in the other way.

To put it in simpler terms, our bodies are meant to be in balance, all the time. We should experience such things as stress, anger, happiness, joy, and everything in between. We should eat the healthy foods that make us feel great, but it's fine to indulge in the other foods that you love, too. As long as you enjoy everything in moderation.

Which brings us to our last number on the list:

The tenth thing you can do to treat and prevent any other candida issues is through your diet. I know I have touched on this a couple of times already, but we are going to take it to the next level in the next chapter and look at how you can actually follow the candida diet, ensuring that this issue is a thing of the past.

Don't panic, I am not going to tell you to get rid of all the foods you love, but I am going to show you how to eat right for your stomach, and how to fix this problem completely.

Not to mention keeping it from coming back again.

Chapter 4 – Candida Diet: Keeping It Real

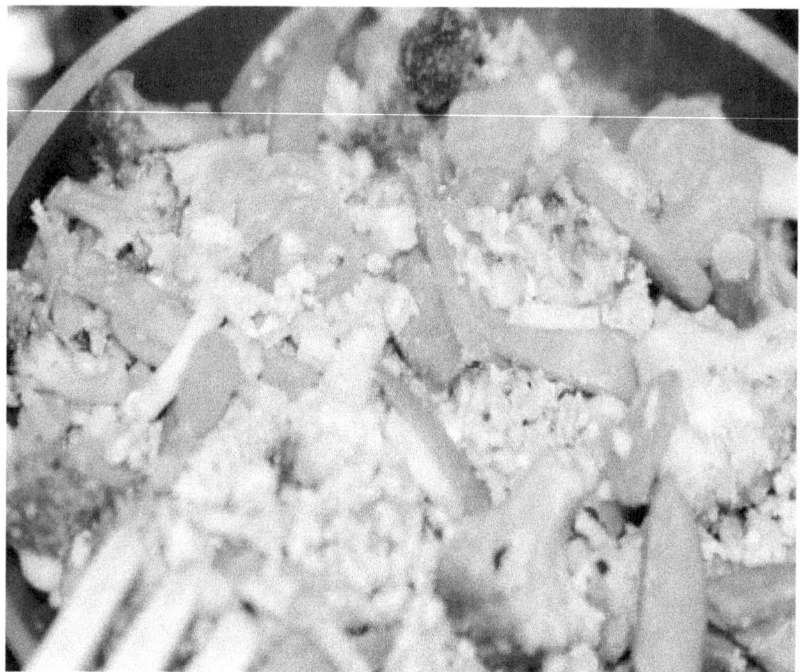

When I make mention to people with this issue that they need to watch their consumption of alcohol, white carbs, and white sugar, they often look at me in horror and ask me what they have left to enjoy.

I know this is the general feeling, especially if you like baked items or a drink every now and then, and I don't want you to think that I am going to take these from you, but I do want to help you stay away from this problem for good, because nothing you eat right now is going to feel as good as getting rid of this problem in your life.

Instead of lining up a strict diet of the things you can have versus the things you can't, I am going to give you a list of the things you can have, you can enjoy moderately, and the things you should modify.

Let's start with the good news, here are the things that you can enjoy on a regular basis, in as much as you want:

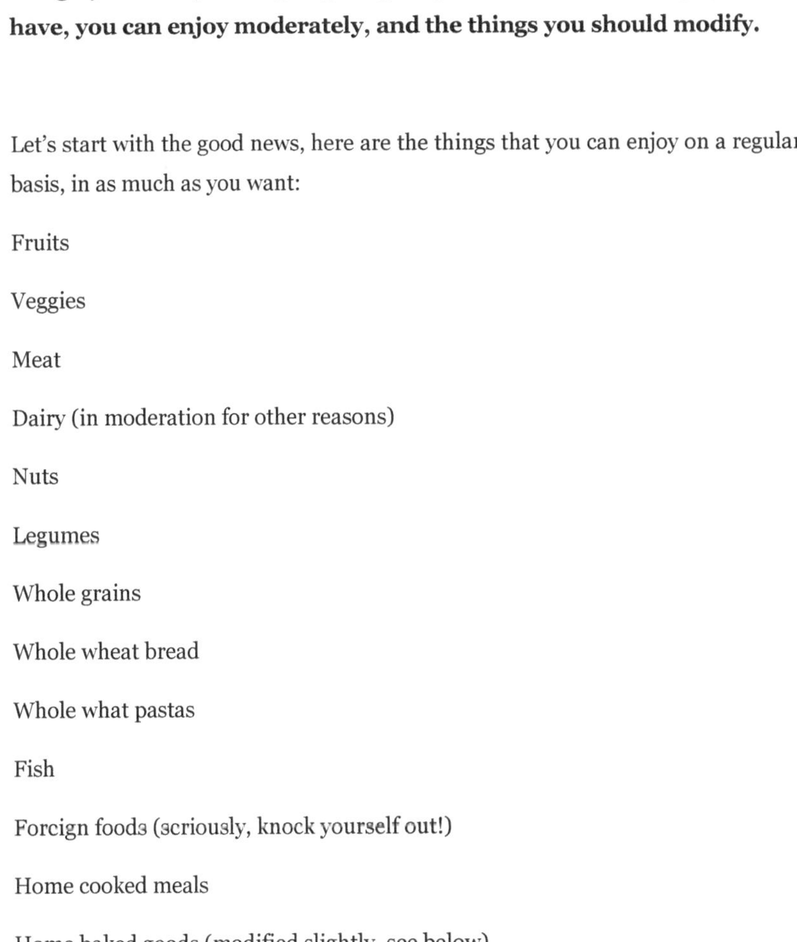

Fruits

Veggies

Meat

Dairy (in moderation for other reasons)

Nuts

Legumes

Whole grains

Whole wheat bread

Whole what pastas

Fish

Forcign foods (scriously, knock yourself out!)

Home cooked meals

Home baked goods (modified slightly, see below)

I know this looks like a short list, but when you think about all the things that are included in this list, you are going to see that you can have just about anything that you had before, so long as you cut back on the carbs and sugars

Which brings us to our next list, which I think you are going to find to be much shorter than the first, and easier to avoid.

White flour products (pastas, breads, baked items)

High sugar items (Sodas, candies, overly sweetened desserts)

Hard alcohol

Processed foods (think things that are prepackaged, whether they are frozen, dehydrated, or anything close to that list. If you only have to open it and enjoy, you may want to think twice about putting it into your body).

As you can see here, this isn't a bad list at all. Sure, there may be some things you have to watch out for, but all in all, you can have the same foods, but you need to have them slightly different than before, or in moderation.

Which is going to bring us to our final list. These are the things you can still have, but you should have in moderation, or you should modify so you can have more of them

Basically, these are the easy swaps you can make in your diet to ensure that you can have the foods you love, but in a way that isn't going to cause you any candida problems

Beer and wine for hard alcohol (again, keep this in moderation)

Swap the white flour for the whole wheat (you will find tons of options at the store)

Skip the sodas as much as possible, or enjoy in highly limited quantities (no more than one or two a week)

Make the same food you love, only make it yourself (don't buy the premade pizzas and casseroles, get the ingredients and make them yourself. This is not only going to cut back on preservatives and excess sugar, it will give you the opportunity to swap white flour and whole wheat as well.)

Then there are the fermented foods.

We all love sauerkraut, kombucha, and those other foods that are good for your gut, but you have to keep in mind that they can have hidden issues such as sugars, salts, or other things that could activate your candida.

All in all, you can enjoy these, but as with anything else, enjoy them in moderation.

Moderation is the key to everything, setting up the perfect balance in your stomach that is going to show everywhere.

Chapter 5 – The Healthy Life: Candida Where it Should Be

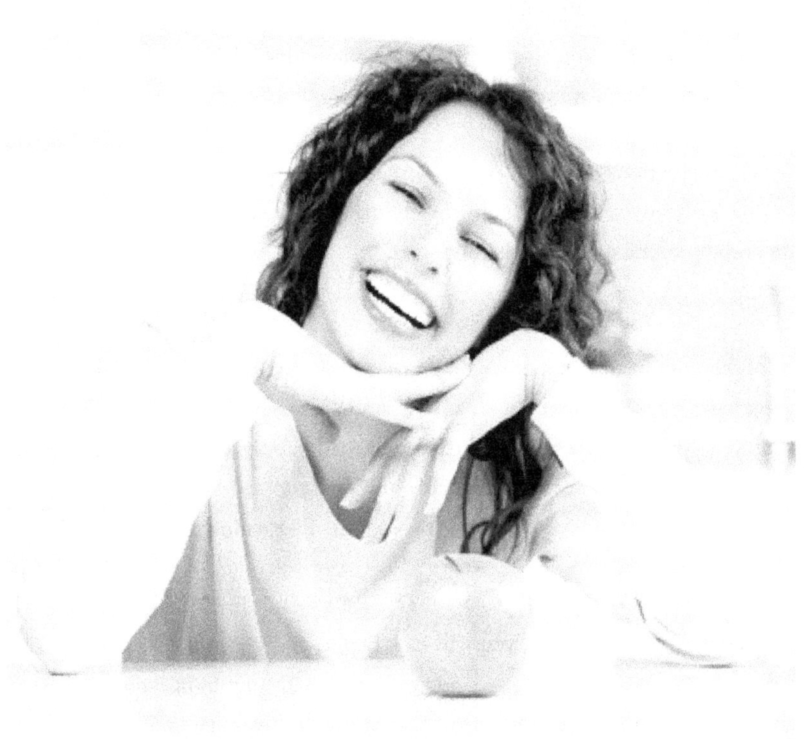

I am sure by now you are feeling a lot better about your candida issue, and you can see that it isn't anything you need to stress about. Sure, you are going to need to make a few changes in your diet, and I highly recommend you get your stress levels under control if you are dealing with that, but overall, this is going to be an easy to way to manage this issue when you do have it, and keep it from coming back later on.

All in all, to keep this from coming back, stick with your diet, and watch out for the sugary foods. Don't fall into the trap of thinking that it is so easy this one time so you may as well do it this way, because that is one of the fastest ways to get caught up in eating ways you shouldn't, and in no time at all you are stuck.

As I have already said, make sure you are drinking plenty of water, and that you are keeping your exercise levels consistent.

All of this combined is not only going to cure your candida problem, but you are going to see so many other benefits in your body as well. As hard as it is to think, candida is an issue that comes when you are out balance in your life, and when you restore that balance, you are not only going to see improvements in the candida issue itself, but you are going to see it in other realms, too.

You are going to feel better, you will look better, and you will be healthier. You will get sick less often, and it is going to help with any indigestion you have experienced. All in all, you may have thought that this was just one issue that you could fix with just one little solution, but the things you are going to be able to fix when you are careful are going to surprise you.

I hope this book was able to show you just how easy it is to change your life, and how you can start with this treatment today. You are going to see the results, and they are going to last for you. There's no way they can't if you are eating this way, and you'll never want to go back again.

Conclusion

There you have it, everything you need to know about candida. What it is, how to treat it, and how to manage it in the future. Can you imagine a life without any of the symptoms you have had to deal with before now?

Can you imagine what it will be like when you don't have to worry about your breath, your tongue, or any of those nasty yeast infections that like to show up when you least expect it? If you follow the simple steps I outlined in this book, those things are all going to be things of the past, and you will never have to worry about any of them again.

I know right now it can be frustrating, and all you want to do is get rid of the problem, but let me assure you, if you stick with it, even when it isn't easy, you are going to get the results that you want, and they are going to stay.

I know yeast infections are no fun. They are embarrassing, they are painful, and they are annoying. When you have one, all you can think about is how uncomfortable it is, and wonder how you can get rid of it. All you want is a little relief, but you don't want to have to deal with the embarrassment of the store to get there.

I have known people who refused to go get the relief they desire because they are embarrassed about the infections, but they shouldn't be. This is a problem that countless people have, but no one should have to live with. With the simple solutions you find in this book, you are going to get rid of the problem for good.

I know you are going to fall in love with these remedies, and find that the diet is so easy to stick with, you aren't going to have any trouble at all doing it. And when you get the results that you want, and never have to deal with this again, you are going to be so relieved you will want to share this with all of your friends.

I hope this book was able to show you that you can get that relief the fast and easy way, and I hope you start today. There is a lot you can do for your health, and you are going to be so much happier when you know you are in control of what is going on.

No stress, no mess, and no more infections!

Life is going to take on a whole new meaning when you don't have to deal with any of that stuff, and that is just the beginning.

So are you ready to get out there and live your life to the fullest? Go for it.

FREE Bonus Reminder

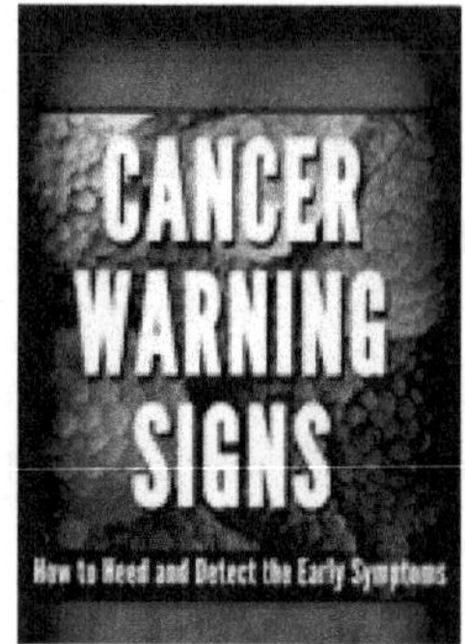

If you have not grabbed it yet, please go ahead and download your special bonus report *"DIY Projects. 13 Useful & Easy To Make DIY Projects To Save Money & Improve Your Home!"*

Simply Click the Button Below

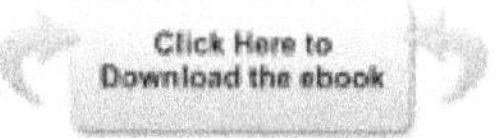

OR Go to This Page

http://healthylivingpeople.com/free/

BONUS #2: More Free & Discounted Books

Do you want to receive more Free & Discounted Books?

We have a mailing list where we send out our new Books when they go free or with a discount on Kindle. Click on the link below to sign up for Free & Discount Book Promotions.

=> **Sign Up for Free & Discount Book Promotions** <=

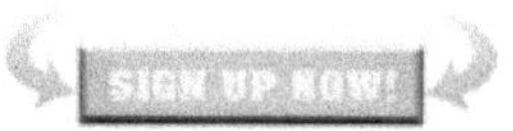

OR Go to this URL